Cultivating Health with Herbal Medicine: The Lost Book of Natural Herbal Remedies A Holistic Approach to Wellness

Contents

Introduction

Welcome to "Cultivating Health with Herbal Medicine: The Lost Book of Natural Herbal Remedies A Holistic Approach to Wellness". In these pages, we embark on a journey through the fascinating world of herbal medicine, exploring its rich history, practical applications, and profound impact on holistic wellness.

Throughout human history, plants have been our companions, providing sustenance, shelter, and healing. Herbal medicine, born from centuries of observation, experimentation, and wisdom passed down through generations, offers a gentle yet potent approach to promoting health and vitality. It is a testament to our enduring relationship with the natural world and our innate capacity for healing.

In this book, we delve into the fundamentals of herbal medicine, from selecting and sourcing herbs to understanding various herbal preparations. We explore the vast array of herbal remedies available for common ailments, from headaches and digestive disorders to stress and skin conditions. Each chapter offers practical insights, empowering you to harness the healing power of plants in your daily life.

But herbal medicine is more than just a collection of remedies—it is a holistic approach to wellness that encompasses mind, body, and spirit. We delve into the interconnectedness of health, exploring how herbal medicine can support detoxification, boost energy levels, and promote long-term health and prevention. Moreover, we examine the integration of herbal medicine with lifestyle practices such as nutrition, mindfulness, and exercise, fostering a holistic approach to well-being.

As you embark on this journey, remember that herbal medicine is a personal path, shaped by individual needs, preferences, and experiences. Whether you are seeking relief from a specific ailment, striving for optimal health, or simply curious about the healing power of plants, may this book serve as a guide and companion on your quest for wellness.

Join me as we rediscover the lost wisdom of natural herbal remedies, cultivating health and vitality with each step along the way.

Welcome to the world of herbal medicine—where nature's pharmacy awaits, ready to nourish, heal, and inspire.

Let's begin.

Chapter 1: The Fundamentals of Herbal Medicine

Herbal medicine, also known as phytotherapy or botanical medicine, is a time-honored practice that utilizes plants and plant extracts for therapeutic purposes. In this chapter, we will delve into the foundational principles of herbal medicine, providing you with a comprehensive understanding of its origins, practices, and applications.

Getting Started with Herbal Medicine: Before delving into the world of herbal medicine, it is essential to understand its fundamental principles and practices. We explore the concept of vitalism—the belief that living organisms possess a vital force or energy that governs health and healing. Herbal medicine operates on the premise that plants contain this vital force, offering a natural source of healing energy.

We will discuss the importance of developing a holistic perspective on health, considering the interconnectedness of mind, body, and spirit. Herbal medicine views health as a dynamic equilibrium, influenced by various factors such as diet, lifestyle, environment, and emotional well-being.

Selecting and Sourcing Herbs: Central to herbal medicine is the selection and sourcing of herbs. We will explore the importance of sourcing high-quality, organically grown herbs to ensure their potency and safety. We discuss the significance of sustainable harvesting practices, emphasizing the need to respect and protect the natural environment.

Additionally, we will provide practical tips for selecting herbs based on their medicinal properties and therapeutic benefits. Understanding the energetics and actions of herbs—such as whether they are warming or cooling, drying or moistening—will empower you to choose the most appropriate herbs for your individual needs.

Understanding Herbal Preparations: Herbal medicine encompasses a wide range of preparations, each with its unique properties and applications. We will explore various methods of preparing and administering herbs, including:

- Infusions and teas: Extracting the medicinal properties of herbs through steeping in hot water.

- Decoctions: Boiling herbs to extract their active constituents, often used for roots, bark, and seeds.

- Tinctures: Extracting herbs in alcohol or glycerin to create concentrated liquid extracts.

- Poultices and compresses: Applying herbs externally to relieve pain, inflammation, or promote healing.

Understanding these different preparations will enable you to choose the most suitable method for administering herbs based on their therapeutic properties and desired effects.

Safety Considerations and Precautions:
While herbal medicine offers many benefits, it is essential to approach it with caution and respect. We will discuss safety considerations and precautions to ensure the responsible use of herbs:

- Understanding potential interactions with medications and existing health conditions.

- Recognizing signs of allergic reactions or adverse effects.

- Consulting with a qualified herbalist or healthcare professional before starting any herbal regimen, especially if pregnant, nursing, or taking medications.

By prioritizing safety and informed decision-making, you can enjoy the benefits of herbal medicine while minimizing potential risks.

Conclusion: In this chapter, we have laid the groundwork for your journey into the world of herbal medicine. By understanding the fundamental principles of herbalism, selecting and sourcing high-quality herbs, mastering various herbal preparations, and prioritizing safety, you are equipped to embark on a path of holistic healing and well-being.

In the chapters that follow, we will explore specific herbal remedies for common ailments, detoxification and cleansing practices, strategies for boosting energy and vitality, and much more. Join us as we unlock the healing power of nature's pharmacy and cultivate health and wellness through the art and science of herbal medicine.

Chapter 2: Herbal Remedies for Common Ailments

In this chapter, we delve into the world of herbal remedies for addressing common ailments that affect many individuals in their daily lives. From headaches to digestive discomforts, sleep disturbances, and stress, herbal medicine offers a natural and effective approach to managing and alleviating these issues. Let's explore a variety of herbal remedies tailored to specific health concerns:

1. **Headaches and Migraines:** Headaches and migraines can be debilitating, impacting daily activities and overall well-being. Herbal remedies such as feverfew,

white willow bark, and peppermint can help alleviate headache symptoms by reducing inflammation, relaxing tense muscles, and promoting circulation. Additionally, incorporating calming herbs like chamomile and lavender into teas or aromatherapy can help soothe tension and promote relaxation.

2. **Digestive Disorders:** Digestive discomforts such as indigestion, gas, and bloating are common complaints that can disrupt daily life. Herbal remedies such as ginger, peppermint, and fennel can help ease digestive symptoms by

promoting digestion, reducing gas, and soothing inflammation. Herbal teas or tinctures containing these herbs can be taken before or after meals to support digestive health.

3. **Sleep Disorders and Insomnia:** Sleep disorders and insomnia can have a profound impact on physical and mental health. Herbal remedies such as valerian root, passionflower, and chamomile have been traditionally used to promote relaxation, reduce anxiety, and improve sleep quality. These herbs can be consumed in tea form or taken as supplements before bedtime to support restful sleep.

4. **Stress and Anxiety Relief:** Stress and anxiety are prevalent in today's fast-paced world, affecting many individuals on a daily basis. Herbal remedies such as holy basil (tulsi), lemon balm, and ashwagandha have adaptogenic properties, helping the body adapt to stress and promote relaxation. Incorporating these herbs into teas, tinctures, or capsules can help support the body's natural stress response and promote emotional well-being.

5. **Respiratory Health:** Respiratory conditions such as coughs, congestion, and asthma can be uncomfortable and disruptive to

daily life. Herbal remedies such as thyme, licorice root, and marshmallow root have expectorant and soothing properties that can help alleviate respiratory symptoms and support lung health. Herbal teas, steam inhalations, or herbal syrups can be effective ways to deliver these remedies directly to the respiratory system.

6. **Skin Conditions:** Skin conditions such as acne, eczema, and psoriasis can be challenging to manage, often requiring a holistic approach to treatment. Herbal remedies such as calendula, burdock root, and aloe vera have anti-inflammatory and

healing properties that can help soothe irritated skin, reduce inflammation, and promote healing. Topical applications such as creams, salves, or poultices containing these herbs can be beneficial for managing skin conditions.

7. **Immune System Support:** Supporting the immune system is essential for overall health and well-being, especially during times of illness or stress. Herbal remedies such as echinacea, elderberry, and astragalus have immune-modulating properties that can help strengthen the body's natural defenses and promote resilience against

infections. These herbs can be consumed as teas, tinctures, or supplements to support immune function.

8. **Women's Health:** Women's health issues such as menstrual cramps, menopause symptoms, and hormonal imbalances can be effectively managed with herbal remedies. Herbs such as black cohosh, dong quai, and red raspberry leaf have been traditionally used to support women's reproductive health and balance hormonal fluctuations. Herbal teas, tinctures, or capsules containing these herbs can help

alleviate menstrual discomfort, hot flashes, and other menopausal symptoms.

9. **Men's Health:** Men's health concerns such as prostate issues, erectile dysfunction, and hormonal imbalances can also benefit from herbal remedies. Herbs such as saw palmetto, tribulus terrestris, and horny goat weed have been traditionally used to support prostate health, improve libido, and balance testosterone levels. These herbs can be consumed as teas, tinctures, or supplements to support men's reproductive health and vitality.

Chapter 3: Herbs for Detoxification and Cleansing

In this chapter, we explore the role of herbal medicine in supporting the body's natural detoxification and cleansing processes. Detoxification is essential for eliminating toxins, metabolic waste, and harmful substances from the body, promoting overall health and well-being. By incorporating specific herbs and practices into your routine, you can support your body's detoxification pathways and enhance vitality. Let's delve into the world of herbal remedies for detoxification and cleansing:

Understanding Detoxification:

Detoxification is a natural process by which the body eliminates toxins and waste products through various organs such as the liver, kidneys, colon, lungs, and skin. However, factors such as poor diet, environmental toxins, stress, and sedentary lifestyles can overload the body's detoxification pathways, leading to toxin accumulation and health imbalances. Herbal medicine offers a holistic approach to supporting detoxification by enhancing the function of these organs and promoting the elimination of toxins from the body.

Herbal Teas and Infusions for Detox:

Herbal teas and infusions are an excellent

way to support the body's detoxification process. Herbs such as dandelion root, milk thistle, burdock root, and nettle leaf have traditionally been used to support liver health and promote detoxification. These herbs contain compounds that stimulate bile production, enhance liver function, and facilitate the elimination of toxins from the body. Drinking herbal teas or infusions containing these herbs can help support liver detoxification and promote overall detoxification processes in the body.

Detoxifying Baths and Poultices: In addition to internal detoxification, external methods such as detoxifying baths and poultices can help promote toxin elimination through the skin. Herbs such as Epsom salt, ginger, lavender, and rosemary can be added to bathwater to create a detoxifying soak that helps draw out toxins through the skin. Similarly, herbal poultices made from herbs such as activated charcoal, bentonite clay, and calendula can be applied topically to draw out impurities and promote skin detoxification.

Liver and Kidney Support: The liver and kidneys play a crucial role in detoxification by filtering and eliminating toxins from the body. Herbal remedies such as milk thistle, dandelion root, artichoke leaf, and parsley have traditionally been used to support liver and kidney health and promote detoxification. These herbs contain compounds that help protect liver cells from damage, enhance liver function, and increase urine flow to facilitate toxin elimination through the kidneys.

Incorporating Detoxifying Herbs into Your Diet: Incorporating detoxifying herbs into your diet is a simple and effective way to support detoxification on a daily basis. You can add detoxifying herbs such as cilantro, parsley, garlic, and turmeric to your meals and recipes to enhance flavor and promote detoxification. Additionally, herbal supplements containing detoxifying herbs can be taken as part of a comprehensive detoxification program to support liver, kidney, and overall detoxification processes in the body.

Conclusion: In this chapter, we have explored the role of herbal medicine in supporting the body's natural detoxification and cleansing processes. By incorporating specific herbs and practices into your routine, you can enhance the function of detoxification organs such as the liver and kidneys, promote toxin elimination, and enhance overall vitality and well-being. Experiment with different herbs and detoxification methods to find what works best for you, and consult with a qualified herbalist or healthcare professional for personalized guidance and recommendations.

Chapter 4: Herbal Remedies for Energy and Vitality

In this chapter, we delve into the realm of herbal remedies specifically tailored to boost energy levels, enhance vitality, and promote overall well-being. In today's fast-paced world, many individuals struggle with fatigue, low energy, and stress, making it essential to explore natural approaches to support energy production and resilience. Let's explore a variety of herbs and practices aimed at revitalizing the body and mind:

Boosting Energy Levels Naturally: Chronic fatigue and low energy levels can significantly impact daily life, leading to decreased productivity and overall well-being. Herbal remedies such as ginseng, rhodiola, and ashwagandha have adaptogenic properties, helping the body adapt to stress, increase energy levels, and enhance resilience. These herbs work by supporting the adrenal glands, balancing cortisol levels, and promoting optimal energy production at the cellular level.

Herbal Adaptogens for Stress Management: Stress is a common underlying factor contributing to fatigue and low energy levels. Herbal adaptogens are a class of herbs that help the body adapt to stress and promote overall resilience. Herbs such as holy basil (tulsi), eleuthero (Siberian ginseng), and licorice root have been traditionally used to support the body's stress response, balance stress hormones, and enhance energy levels. Incorporating adaptogenic herbs into your daily routine can help increase energy, reduce fatigue, and improve overall well-being.

Enhancing Mental Clarity and Focus: Mental fatigue and lack of focus are common challenges in today's information-driven society. Herbal remedies such as ginkgo biloba, gotu kola, and bacopa have cognitive-enhancing properties, promoting mental clarity, focus, and cognitive function. These herbs work by increasing blood flow to the brain, supporting neurotransmitter function, and protecting brain cells from oxidative damage. Incorporating these herbs into your daily regimen can help enhance cognitive performance, improve memory, and support overall brain health.

Nourishing and Rejuvenating Herbs: Herbal tonics and nutritive herbs are a valuable ally in promoting long-term energy and vitality. Herbs such as nettle leaf, oatstraw, and red clover are rich in vitamins, minerals, and antioxidants, nourishing the body and supporting overall vitality. These herbs work by replenishing essential nutrients, supporting adrenal health, and promoting systemic balance. Incorporating herbal tonics and nutritive herbs into your diet can help replenish energy reserves, enhance vitality, and support overall well-being.

Holistic Lifestyle Practices for Energy: In addition to herbal remedies, holistic lifestyle practices play a crucial role in supporting energy and vitality. Practices such as regular exercise, adequate sleep, stress management, and a balanced diet are essential for maintaining optimal energy levels and overall well-being. Incorporating mindfulness techniques such as meditation, yoga, and deep breathing exercises can also help reduce stress, increase energy, and promote mental clarity and focus.

Conclusion: In this chapter, we have explored a variety of herbal remedies and practices aimed at boosting energy levels, enhancing vitality, and promoting overall well-being. By incorporating adaptogenic herbs, cognitive-enhancing herbs, nourishing tonics, and holistic lifestyle practices into your daily routine, you can support optimal energy production, reduce fatigue, and enhance resilience in the face of stress and challenges. Experiment with different herbs and practices to find what works best for you, and consult with a qualified herbalist or healthcare professional for personalized guidance and recommendations.

Chapter 5: Herbal Remedies for Long-Term Health and Prevention

In this chapter, we explore the use of herbal medicine as a proactive approach to promoting long-term health, preventing illness, and supporting overall well-being. Rather than simply addressing symptoms as they arise, herbal remedies can be used strategically to nourish and strengthen the body, enhance resilience, and reduce the risk of chronic disease. Let's delve into a variety of herbs and practices aimed at supporting long-term health and prevention:

Anti-inflammatory Herbs for Chronic Conditions: Chronic inflammation is a common underlying factor in many health conditions, including heart disease, diabetes, arthritis, and autoimmune disorders. Herbal remedies such as turmeric, ginger, and boswellia have potent anti-inflammatory properties, helping to reduce inflammation, ease pain, and support overall health. These herbs work by inhibiting inflammatory pathways, modulating the immune response, and protecting against oxidative stress.

Heart Health and Circulation Support: Maintaining cardiovascular health is essential for overall well-being and longevity. Herbal remedies such as hawthorn, garlic, and motherwort have traditionally been used to support heart health, improve circulation, and reduce the risk of heart disease. These herbs work by promoting healthy blood pressure, cholesterol levels, and blood flow to the heart and blood vessels. Incorporating heart-healthy herbs into your daily regimen can help support cardiovascular function and reduce the risk of heart-related complications.

Joint and Muscle Pain Relief: Joint and muscle pain can significantly impact mobility and quality of life, especially as we age. Herbal remedies such as devil's claw, white willow bark, and arnica have analgesic and anti-inflammatory properties, helping to relieve pain, reduce inflammation, and improve joint mobility. These herbs work by inhibiting pain pathways, reducing inflammation, and promoting tissue healing. Incorporating herbal remedies for joint and muscle pain into your routine can help alleviate discomfort and support mobility and flexibility.

Cognitive Health and Memory Enhancement: Maintaining cognitive health and sharp mental acuity is essential for overall well-being and quality of life. Herbal remedies such as ginkgo biloba, bacopa, and rosemary have cognitive-enhancing properties, supporting memory, concentration, and mental clarity. These herbs work by increasing blood flow to the brain, enhancing neurotransmitter function, and protecting brain cells from oxidative damage. Incorporating cognitive-enhancing herbs into your daily regimen can help support cognitive function and reduce the risk of age-related cognitive decline.

Immune System Support: Supporting a healthy immune system is crucial for preventing illness and maintaining overall health and vitality. Herbal remedies such as echinacea, elderberry, and astragalus have immune-modulating properties, helping to strengthen the body's natural defenses and reduce the risk of infections. These herbs work by stimulating immune cell activity, enhancing antibody production, and supporting overall immune function. Incorporating immune-supportive herbs into your daily routine can help bolster your body's defenses and promote resilience against pathogens.

Conclusion: In this chapter, we have explored the use of herbal medicine as a proactive approach to promoting long-term health and preventing illness. By incorporating anti-inflammatory herbs, heart-healthy herbs, joint and muscle pain remedies, cognitive-enhancing herbs, and immune-supportive herbs into your daily regimen, you can support overall well-being, reduce the risk of chronic disease, and enhance vitality and resilience. Experiment with different herbs and practices to find what works best for you, and consult with a qualified herbalist or healthcare professional for personalized guidance and recommendations.

Chapter 6: Creating Your Herbal Medicine Cabinet

In this chapter, we embark on the journey of creating and maintaining your herbal medicine cabinet—a personalized collection of herbs, remedies, and tools to support your health and well-being. From establishing a home apothecary to storing and preserving herbs, we'll explore the practical aspects of herbal medicine preparation and usage.

Establishing a Home Herbal Apothecary: A home herbal apothecary serves as the foundation of your herbal medicine practice. Begin by selecting a designated space in your home—a shelf, cupboard, or drawer—to store your herbs and supplies. Invest in glass jars, bottles, and containers to store dried herbs, tinctures, and herbal preparations. Consider labeling each container with the herb's name, date of purchase, and expiration date to ensure freshness and potency.

Selecting and Sourcing Herbs: When selecting herbs for your apothecary, prioritize high-quality, organically grown herbs to ensure their potency and purity. Choose reputable suppliers and sources that prioritize sustainable harvesting practices and ethical sourcing. Consider growing your own herbs in a garden or indoor containers to have a fresh and readily available supply of herbs for your remedies.

Storing and Preserving Herbs: Proper storage and preservation are essential for maintaining the potency and freshness of your herbs. Store dried herbs in airtight containers away from direct sunlight, heat, and moisture to prevent degradation. Consider using dark glass jars or opaque containers to protect herbs from light exposure. Store liquid herbal preparations such as tinctures and infused oils in amber glass bottles to protect them from light and oxidation.

DIY Herbal Remedies and Recipes: Experimenting with DIY herbal remedies is a rewarding way to harness the healing power of plants. Stock your herbal medicine cabinet with essential supplies such as carrier oils, beeswax, and herbs for creating homemade salves, balms, and ointments. Explore herbal tea blends for relaxation, immune support, and digestive health. Experiment with herbal tinctures, syrups, and elixirs for targeted support of specific health concerns.

Herbal Medicine Preparation Methods: Familiarize yourself with various herbal medicine preparation methods, including infusions, decoctions, tinctures, and poultices. Infusions involve steeping herbs in hot water to extract their medicinal properties, while decoctions involve boiling herbs to extract their active constituents. Tinctures are concentrated liquid extracts of herbs made by macerating herbs in alcohol or glycerin. Poultices involve applying mashed or powdered herbs directly to the skin for localized relief.

Safety Considerations and Precautions: Prioritize safety and responsible usage when working with herbs and herbal remedies. Research potential contraindications, interactions, and precautions associated with specific herbs, especially if you are pregnant, nursing, or taking medications. Start with small doses when trying new herbs and monitor for any adverse reactions. Consult with a qualified herbalist or healthcare professional for personalized guidance and recommendations.

Conclusion: In this chapter, we have explored the practical aspects of creating and maintaining your herbal medicine cabinet. By establishing a home apothecary, selecting high-quality herbs, storing and preserving herbs properly, and experimenting with DIY herbal remedies, you can empower yourself to take charge of your health and well-being with the healing power of plants. Remember to prioritize safety and responsible usage when working with herbs, and consult with a qualified herbalist or healthcare professional for personalized guidance and recommendations.

Chapter 7: Holistic Lifestyle Practices

In this chapter, we delve into the integration of herbal medicine with holistic lifestyle practices, emphasizing the importance of nurturing mind, body, and spirit for optimal health and well-being. By incorporating mindfulness, nutrition, movement, and stress management techniques into your daily routine, you can synergize the benefits of herbal medicine and cultivate a balanced and vibrant life.

Integrating Herbal Medicine with Diet and Nutrition: Nutrition forms the foundation of health, providing essential nutrients and energy for bodily functions.

Integrate herbal medicine with a balanced diet rich in whole foods, fruits, vegetables, and lean proteins to support overall health and well-being. Incorporate nutrient-dense herbs such as parsley, cilantro, and dandelion greens into your meals to boost flavor and nutritional value. Experiment with herbal teas, infusions, and culinary herbs to enhance digestion, support immune function, and promote vitality.

Mindfulness and Meditation for Wellness: Cultivating mindfulness and meditation practices can have profound benefits for mental and emotional well-being. Set aside time each day for meditation, deep breathing exercises, or mindfulness practices to reduce stress, enhance self-awareness, and promote relaxation. Incorporate calming herbs such as chamomile, lemon balm, and lavender into your meditation routine to deepen relaxation and promote inner peace.

Exercise and Movement for Vitality: Regular physical activity is essential for maintaining overall health and vitality. Find activities that you enjoy, whether it's walking, yoga, dancing, or gardening, and incorporate them into your daily routine. Herbal remedies such as ginseng, rhodiola, and maca root can help support energy levels, endurance, and recovery during physical activity. Prioritize movement and exercise as part of your holistic lifestyle to promote cardiovascular health, maintain muscle tone, and enhance overall well-being.

Stress Management Techniques: Chronic stress can have detrimental effects on physical and mental health, contributing to a wide range of health issues. Explore stress management techniques such as deep breathing exercises, progressive muscle relaxation, and guided imagery to promote relaxation and reduce stress levels. Herbal adaptogens such as ashwagandha, holy basil (tulsi), and rhodiola can help support the body's stress response, balance cortisol levels, and promote resilience during times of stress. Prioritize self-care and stress management as essential components of your holistic lifestyle to enhance overall well-being and vitality.

Cultivating Connection with Nature: Connecting with nature is essential for grounding, rejuvenation, and overall well-being. Spend time outdoors in natural settings, such as parks, forests, or gardens, to reconnect with the rhythms of the earth and nourish your spirit. Herbal remedies such as pine needle tea, forest bathing, and herbal gardening can deepen your connection with nature and promote a sense of harmony and balance. Prioritize spending time in nature as part of your holistic lifestyle to nurture your body, mind, and soul.

Conclusion: In this chapter, we have explored the integration of herbal medicine with holistic lifestyle practices to promote overall health and well-being. By incorporating mindfulness, nutrition, movement, stress management techniques, and connection with nature into your daily routine, you can synergize the benefits of herbal medicine and cultivate a balanced and vibrant life. Experiment with different practices and techniques to find what works best for you, and prioritize self-care as an essential component of your holistic lifestyle journey.

Chapter 8: Herbal Remedies for Digestive Health

In this chapter, we delve into the realm of herbal remedies specifically tailored to support digestive health—a key aspect of overall well-being. The digestive system plays a crucial role in nutrient absorption, waste elimination, and immune function, making it essential to maintain its optimal function. Let's explore a variety of herbs and practices aimed at promoting digestive comfort, supporting gastrointestinal function, and enhancing overall digestive wellness:

Managing Irritable Bowel Syndrome (IBS): Irritable Bowel Syndrome (IBS) is a common digestive disorder characterized by abdominal pain, bloating, gas, and changes in bowel habits. Herbal remedies such as peppermint, chamomile, and fennel can help alleviate symptoms of IBS by reducing intestinal spasms, soothing inflammation, and promoting digestion. Drinking herbal teas containing these herbs can provide relief from discomfort and support overall digestive health.

Herbal Remedies for Acid Reflux: Acid reflux, also known as gastroesophageal reflux disease (GERD), occurs when stomach acid flows back into the esophagus, causing heartburn and discomfort. Herbal remedies such as licorice root, marshmallow root, and slippery elm bark can help soothe irritated mucous membranes, reduce inflammation, and protect the esophagus from acid damage. Consuming herbal teas or supplements containing these herbs before meals can help alleviate symptoms of acid reflux and support digestive comfort.

Relieving Constipation Naturally: Constipation is a common digestive complaint characterized by infrequent bowel movements and difficulty passing stool. Herbal remedies such as senna, cascara sagrada, and aloe vera have natural laxative properties that can help stimulate bowel movements and relieve constipation. However, it's essential to use these herbs judiciously and under the guidance of a healthcare professional to prevent dependency and maintain digestive balance.

Supporting Gut Health with Probiotic Herbs: Maintaining a healthy balance of gut bacteria is essential for overall digestive health and immune function. Probiotic herbs such as dandelion root, burdock root, and chicory root contain prebiotic fibers that help nourish beneficial gut bacteria and support gut flora balance. Incorporating these herbs into your diet or consuming them as herbal teas can help promote digestive wellness and support immune function.

Herbs for Digestive Comfort: In addition to addressing specific digestive issues, certain herbs can help promote overall digestive comfort and well-being. Herbs such as ginger, peppermint, and chamomile have carminative properties that can help reduce gas, bloating, and indigestion. Consuming herbal teas containing these herbs after meals can aid digestion, soothe discomfort, and promote overall digestive wellness.

Conclusion: In this chapter, we have explored a variety of herbal remedies for promoting digestive health and well-being. By incorporating herbs that support digestion, soothe discomfort, and promote gut health into your daily routine, you can enhance overall digestive wellness and improve quality of life. Experiment with different herbs and formulations to find what works best for you, and consult with a qualified herbalist or healthcare professional for personalized guidance and recommendations. Prioritize digestive health as an essential component of your holistic wellness journey, and enjoy the benefits of a happy and healthy digestive system.

Chapter 9: Herbal Remedies for Stress Relief and Emotional Well-Being

In this chapter, we explore the profound impact of herbal medicine on managing stress, promoting relaxation, and supporting emotional well-being. In today's fast-paced world, stress has become a prevalent issue, affecting mental, emotional, and physical health. Herbal remedies offer gentle and effective solutions for managing stress, calming the mind, and fostering a sense of balance and tranquility. Let's delve into a variety of herbs and practices aimed at promoting stress relief and emotional well-being:

Understanding the Impact of Stress on Health: Chronic stress can have far-reaching effects on health, contributing to a wide range of physical and mental health issues, including anxiety, depression, insomnia, digestive disorders, and cardiovascular disease. Understanding the impact of stress on health is the first step in addressing its underlying causes and implementing effective stress management strategies.

Herbal Adaptogens for Stress Resilience: Adaptogenic herbs are a class of herbs that help the body adapt to stress and promote overall resilience. Herbs such as ashwagandha, holy basil (tulsi), and rhodiola have adaptogenic properties, helping to balance stress hormones, support adrenal function, and promote relaxation. Incorporating adaptogenic herbs into your daily routine can help increase resilience to stress, reduce anxiety, and enhance overall well-being.

Calming Nervine Herbs for Relaxation: Nervine herbs are herbs that have a calming and soothing effect on the nervous system, promoting relaxation and reducing anxiety. Herbs such as chamomile, lemon balm, and passionflower have nervine properties, helping to calm the mind, reduce tension, and promote restful sleep. Consuming herbal teas or tinctures containing these herbs can help alleviate stress and promote emotional well-being.

Mood-Enhancing Herbs for Emotional Balance: Certain herbs have mood-enhancing properties that can help promote emotional balance and well-being. Herbs such as St. John's wort, lavender, and skullcap have been traditionally used to uplift mood, reduce feelings of sadness and anxiety, and promote a sense of calmness and contentment. Incorporating these herbs into your daily routine can help support emotional resilience and improve overall mood and outlook.

Aromatherapy for Stress Relief: Aromatherapy, the use of essential oils derived from aromatic plants, is a powerful tool for promoting relaxation and stress relief. Essential oils such as lavender, bergamot, and frankincense have calming and soothing properties that can help reduce stress, anxiety, and tension. Diffusing essential oils, adding them to bathwater, or using them in massage oils can help create a calming atmosphere and promote emotional well-being.

Mindfulness Practices for Stress Reduction: In addition to herbal remedies, mindfulness practices such as meditation, deep breathing exercises, and yoga can help reduce stress, promote relaxation, and foster emotional well-being. Set aside time each day for mindfulness practices to quiet the mind, reduce anxiety, and cultivate a sense of inner peace. Incorporating herbal teas or tinctures into your mindfulness routine can enhance relaxation and deepen the therapeutic effects of your practice.

Conclusion: In this chapter, we have explored a variety of herbal remedies and practices for managing stress, promoting relaxation, and supporting emotional well-being. By incorporating adaptogenic herbs, nervine herbs, mood-enhancing herbs, aromatherapy, and mindfulness practices into your daily routine, you can effectively manage stress, reduce anxiety, and foster a sense of balance and tranquility in your life. Experiment with different herbs and practices to find what works best for you, and prioritize self-care as an essential component of your holistic wellness journey.

Chapter 10: Herbal Remedies for Sleep Support and Insomnia Relief

In this chapter, we explore the role of herbal medicine in promoting restful sleep, alleviating insomnia, and enhancing overall sleep quality. Quality sleep is essential for physical, mental, and emotional well-being, yet many individuals struggle with sleep disturbances and insomnia due to various factors such as stress, lifestyle, and underlying health conditions. Herbal remedies offer gentle and effective solutions for improving sleep patterns, calming the mind, and promoting relaxation. Let's delve into a variety of herbs and practices aimed at supporting sleep health and insomnia relief:

Understanding the Importance of Quality Sleep: Quality sleep is crucial for overall health and well-being, supporting various bodily functions such as immune function, hormone regulation, cognitive function, and emotional stability. Lack of sleep or poor sleep quality can have detrimental effects on physical and mental health, leading to increased risk of chronic diseases, impaired cognitive function, mood disturbances, and decreased quality of life. Understanding the importance of quality sleep is the first step in addressing sleep issues and implementing effective sleep support strategies.

Herbal Sedatives for Sleep Promotion: Certain herbs have sedative properties that can help promote relaxation, calm the mind, and induce sleep. Herbs such as valerian root, passionflower, and California poppy have been traditionally used to alleviate insomnia, reduce anxiety, and improve sleep quality. Consuming herbal teas, tinctures, or capsules containing these herbs before bedtime can help facilitate the onset of sleep and promote restful sleep throughout the night.

Nervine Herbs for Stress Reduction: Stress and anxiety are common contributors to sleep disturbances and insomnia. Nervine herbs are herbs that have a calming and soothing effect on the nervous system, helping to reduce tension, anxiety, and restlessness. Herbs such as chamomile, lemon balm, and skullcap have nervine properties that can help promote relaxation, reduce stress, and prepare the body and mind for sleep. Incorporating nervine herbs into your bedtime routine can help calm the mind and promote a sense of tranquility conducive to restful sleep.

Aromatherapy for Sleep Support: Aromatherapy, the use of essential oils derived from aromatic plants, is a powerful tool for promoting relaxation and sleep support. Essential oils such as lavender, roman chamomile, and cedarwood have calming and sedative properties that can help promote relaxation, reduce anxiety, and improve sleep quality. Diffusing these essential oils in the bedroom, adding them to a warm bath, or applying them topically as part of a bedtime ritual can help create a soothing environment conducive to restful sleep.

Lifestyle Practices for Sleep Hygiene: In addition to herbal remedies, adopting healthy lifestyle practices can help promote sleep hygiene and improve sleep quality. Establish a regular sleep schedule by going to bed and waking up at the same time each day, even on weekends. Create a relaxing bedtime routine that includes activities such as reading, gentle stretching, or listening to calming music to signal to your body that it's time to wind down. Avoid stimulating activities, caffeine, and electronic devices close to bedtime, as they can interfere with sleep onset and quality.

Conclusion: In this chapter, we have explored a variety of herbal remedies and practices for promoting restful sleep, alleviating insomnia, and enhancing overall sleep quality. By incorporating sedative herbs, nervine herbs, aromatherapy, and healthy sleep hygiene practices into your bedtime routine, you can effectively manage sleep disturbances and improve sleep patterns. Experiment with different herbs and practices to find what works best for you, and prioritize sleep as an essential component of your holistic wellness journey. With the gentle support of herbal medicine and lifestyle practices, you can enjoy restorative sleep and wake up feeling refreshed and rejuvenated each day.

Chapter 11: Herbal Remedies for Respiratory Health

In this chapter, we explore the use of herbal medicine in supporting respiratory health—a vital aspect of overall well-being, particularly in today's world where respiratory issues are increasingly common. From coughs and colds to allergies and asthma, the respiratory system can be susceptible to a variety of challenges. Herbal remedies offer natural and effective solutions for supporting respiratory function, soothing irritation, and promoting lung health. Let's delve into a variety of herbs and practices aimed at supporting respiratory health:

Understanding Respiratory Health: The respiratory system plays a crucial role in delivering oxygen to the body and removing carbon dioxide, making it essential for overall health and vitality. Respiratory issues such as coughs, colds, allergies, and asthma can impact breathing, energy levels, and quality of life. Understanding the importance of respiratory health is the first step in addressing respiratory issues and implementing effective support strategies.

Herbal Expectorants for Mucus Clearance: Excessive mucus production can lead to congestion and difficulty breathing, particularly during respiratory infections. Herbal expectorants such as thyme, licorice root, and elecampane help promote the clearance of mucus from the respiratory tract, making it easier to breathe and reducing coughing. Consuming herbal teas or tinctures containing these herbs can help alleviate congestion and support respiratory comfort during colds and flu.

Soothing Demulcent Herbs for Irritation: Irritation of the respiratory tract can cause coughing, throat soreness, and discomfort. Demulcent herbs such as marshmallow root, slippery elm bark, and mullein have soothing properties that help coat and protect the mucous membranes of the respiratory tract, reducing irritation and promoting healing. Consuming herbal teas or lozenges containing these herbs can help soothe a sore throat and alleviate coughing.

Herbal Bronchodilators for Airway Support: Bronchodilators are substances that help relax and open up the airways, making it easier to breathe, particularly for individuals with asthma or bronchitis. Herbal bronchodilators such as eucalyptus, peppermint, and lobelia have been traditionally used to support respiratory function and promote bronchial relaxation. Inhaling steam infused with these essential oils or using herbal inhalers can help provide relief from respiratory congestion and support lung health.

Immune-Modulating Herbs for Respiratory Support: Supporting the immune system is essential for overall respiratory health, particularly during times of illness or seasonal allergies. Immune-modulating herbs such as echinacea, elderberry, and astragalus help strengthen the body's natural defenses and reduce the risk of respiratory infections. Consuming herbal teas, tinctures, or supplements containing these herbs can help support immune function and promote respiratory wellness.

Lifestyle Practices for Respiratory Wellness: In addition to herbal remedies, adopting healthy lifestyle practices can help promote respiratory wellness. Avoiding exposure to environmental pollutants, quitting smoking, staying hydrated, and practicing good hygiene habits can all help support respiratory function and reduce the risk of respiratory infections. Regular exercise, deep breathing exercises, and maintaining a healthy diet rich in fruits, vegetables, and antioxidants can also help support lung health and overall well-being.

Conclusion: In this chapter, we have explored a variety of herbal remedies and practices for supporting respiratory health. By incorporating expectorant herbs, demulcent herbs, bronchodilators, immune-modulating herbs, and healthy lifestyle practices into your daily routine, you can effectively support respiratory function, soothe irritation, and promote lung health. Experiment with different herbs and practices to find what works best for you, and prioritize respiratory health as an essential component of your holistic wellness journey. With the gentle support of herbal medicine and lifestyle practices, you can breathe easier and enjoy optimal respiratory wellness.

Chapter 12: Herbal Remedies for Skin Health and Beauty

In this chapter, we explore the diverse array of herbal remedies available to support skin health and enhance natural beauty. Our skin is the largest organ of the body, serving as a protective barrier against environmental toxins and pathogens. From acne and eczema to aging and sun damage, our skin can face a multitude of challenges. Herbal remedies offer gentle and effective solutions for addressing various skin concerns, promoting healing, and enhancing skin radiance. Let's delve into a variety of herbs and practices aimed at supporting skin health and beauty:

Understanding Skin Health: Healthy skin is a reflection of overall well-being, with factors such as diet, lifestyle, and environmental exposures influencing its appearance and function. Skin issues such as acne, eczema, psoriasis, and premature aging can impact self-confidence and quality of life. Understanding the importance of skin health is the first step in adopting a holistic approach to caring for your skin.

Herbal Remedies for Acne and Blemishes: Acne is a common skin condition characterized by the presence of pimples, blackheads, and whiteheads, often caused by factors such as hormonal imbalances, excess sebum production, and bacterial overgrowth. Herbal remedies such as tea tree oil, witch hazel, and calendula have antimicrobial and anti-inflammatory properties that can help reduce acne lesions, soothe inflammation, and promote healing. Incorporating herbal skincare products containing these ingredients into your daily routine can help manage acne and prevent breakouts.

Soothing Herbs for Eczema and Irritated Skin: Eczema is a chronic skin condition characterized by inflammation, itching, and redness, often triggered by factors such as allergies, stress, and environmental irritants. Herbal remedies such as chamomile, oatmeal, and calendula have soothing and anti-inflammatory properties that can help calm irritated skin, reduce itching, and promote healing. Applying herbal creams, lotions, or ointments containing these ingredients can provide relief from eczema symptoms and support skin barrier function.

Anti-Aging Herbs for Youthful Skin: As we age, our skin undergoes changes such as decreased collagen production, loss of elasticity, and increased susceptibility to wrinkles and fine lines. Herbal remedies such as rosehip seed oil, gotu kola, and green tea extract have antioxidant and anti-aging properties that can help protect against free radical damage, stimulate collagen synthesis, and promote skin renewal. Incorporating herbal serums, moisturizers, or facial masks containing these ingredients into your skincare routine can help maintain youthful skin and reduce the signs of aging.

Herbal Sun Protection and After-Sun Care: Excessive sun exposure can lead to sunburn, premature aging, and increased risk of skin cancer. Herbal remedies such as aloe vera gel, coconut oil, and lavender essential oil have soothing and hydrating properties that can help relieve sunburn, reduce inflammation, and promote skin repair. Applying herbal after-sun products containing these ingredients can provide relief from sunburn and support skin recovery after sun exposure.

Herbal Hair and Scalp Care: In addition to skincare, herbal remedies can also support hair and scalp health. Herbs such as rosemary, lavender, and nettle have been traditionally used to promote hair growth, reduce dandruff, and improve scalp circulation. Incorporating herbal hair rinses, oils, or masks containing these herbs into your hair care routine can help nourish and strengthen your hair, leaving it shiny, healthy, and vibrant.

Conclusion: In this chapter, we have explored a variety of herbal remedies and practices for supporting skin health and enhancing natural beauty. By incorporating herbs that address specific skin concerns, promote healing, and protect against environmental damage into your skincare routine, you can achieve radiant and healthy-looking skin. Experiment with different herbs and skincare products to find what works best for you, and prioritize skin health as an essential component of your holistic wellness journey. With the gentle support of herbal medicine, you can nourish and rejuvenate your skin from the inside out, embracing your natural beauty and glowing with confidence.

Chapter 13: Herbal Remedies for Women's Health

In this chapter, we explore the diverse range of herbal remedies available to support women's health throughout various stages of life. From menstrual discomfort and hormonal imbalances to pregnancy and menopause, women's bodies undergo unique physiological changes that can benefit from the gentle and holistic support of herbal medicine. Let's delve into a variety of herbs and practices aimed at promoting women's health and well-being:

Understanding Women's Health: Women's health encompasses a broad spectrum of physical, emotional, and reproductive concerns, influenced by factors such as hormones, lifestyle, and genetics. Conditions such as menstrual irregularities, PMS, fertility issues, and menopausal symptoms can impact quality of life and overall well-being. Understanding the unique needs of women's health is essential for addressing these concerns and implementing effective support strategies.

Herbal Remedies for Menstrual Comfort: Many women experience menstrual discomfort such as cramps, bloating, and mood swings during their monthly cycle. Herbal remedies such as chasteberry (Vitex), dong quai, and cramp bark have been traditionally used to regulate menstrual cycles, reduce pain and inflammation, and balance hormones. Consuming herbal teas, tinctures, or capsules containing these herbs can help alleviate menstrual discomfort and promote hormonal balance.

Supporting Hormonal Balance: Hormonal imbalances can lead to a variety of symptoms such as acne, mood swings, and irregular periods. Herbal remedies such as black cohosh, red clover, and wild yam have hormone-balancing properties that can help regulate menstrual cycles, alleviate PMS symptoms, and support overall hormonal health. Incorporating these herbs into your daily routine can help promote hormonal balance and reduce symptoms associated with hormonal fluctuations.

Herbal Support for Fertility: For women trying to conceive, herbal remedies can offer support for reproductive health and fertility. Herbs such as vitex (chasteberry), red raspberry leaf, and maca root have been traditionally used to regulate menstrual cycles, support ovulation, and improve fertility. Consuming herbal teas, tinctures, or supplements containing these herbs can help enhance reproductive function and optimize fertility.

Herbal Support during Pregnancy: Pregnancy is a time of significant physiological changes, and herbal medicine can offer gentle support for both the mother and the developing baby. Herbs such as ginger, raspberry leaf, and nettle are commonly used during pregnancy to alleviate nausea, support uterine tone, and provide essential nutrients. However, it's essential to consult with a healthcare provider or qualified herbalist before using herbs during pregnancy to ensure safety and appropriateness.

Herbal Support for Menopausal Symptoms: Menopause is a natural transition in a woman's life marked by hormonal changes and symptoms such as hot flashes, night sweats, and mood swings. Herbal remedies such as black cohosh, evening primrose oil, and sage have been traditionally used to alleviate menopausal symptoms, support hormonal balance, and promote overall well-being during this transition. Incorporating these herbs into your daily routine can help manage menopausal symptoms and support a smooth transition through this life stage.

Conclusion: In this chapter, we have explored a variety of herbal remedies and practices for supporting women's health throughout various stages of life. By incorporating herbs that address specific concerns such as menstrual discomfort, hormonal imbalances, fertility issues, pregnancy, and menopause into your daily routine, you can promote women's health and well-being naturally. Experiment with different herbs and formulations to find what works best for you, and prioritize self-care as an essential component of your holistic wellness journey as a woman. With the gentle support of herbal medicine, you can navigate the unique challenges and transitions of womanhood with grace and vitality.

Chapter 14: Herbal Remedies for Men's Health

In this chapter, we explore the diverse range of herbal remedies available to support men's health, addressing specific concerns and promoting overall well-being throughout various stages of life. From prostate health and hormonal balance to vitality and reproductive function, men's bodies undergo unique physiological changes that can benefit from the holistic support of herbal medicine. Let's delve into a variety of herbs and practices aimed at promoting men's health and vitality:

Understanding Men's Health: Men's health encompasses a wide range of physical, emotional, and reproductive concerns, influenced by factors such as hormones, lifestyle, and genetics. Conditions such as prostate enlargement, erectile dysfunction, low testosterone levels, and stress-related issues can impact quality of life and overall well-being. Understanding the unique needs of men's health is essential for addressing these concerns and implementing effective support strategies.

Herbal Support for Prostate Health: Prostate enlargement, also known as benign prostatic hyperplasia (BPH), is a common concern among aging men, often leading to urinary symptoms such as frequent urination and difficulty emptying the bladder. Herbal remedies such as saw palmetto, pygeum bark, and stinging nettle have been traditionally used to support prostate health, reduce inflammation, and alleviate urinary symptoms associated with BPH. Consuming herbal supplements or teas containing these herbs can help support prostate function and promote urinary tract health.

Herbal Support for Hormonal Balance: Hormonal imbalances can affect men's health, leading to symptoms such as low energy, reduced muscle mass, and decreased libido. Herbal remedies such as ashwagandha, tongkat ali, and tribulus terrestris have adaptogenic and aphrodisiac properties that can help balance hormones, increase testosterone levels, and support overall vitality and virility. Incorporating these herbs into your daily routine can help promote hormonal balance and enhance men's health and well-being.

Herbal Support for Erectile Function: Erectile dysfunction (ED) is a common concern among men, characterized by the inability to achieve or maintain an erection sufficient for sexual intercourse. Herbal remedies such as horny goat weed, ginkgo biloba, and Korean red ginseng have been traditionally used to support erectile function, improve blood flow to the genitals, and enhance sexual performance. Consuming herbal supplements or tinctures containing these herbs can help support erectile function and promote sexual vitality.

Herbal Support for Stress Management: Stress can have a significant impact on men's health, affecting hormone levels, immune function, and overall well-being. Herbal adaptogens such as rhodiola, holy basil (tulsi), and Siberian ginseng help the body adapt to stress, increase resilience, and promote energy and vitality. Incorporating these herbs into your daily routine can help support stress management, reduce fatigue, and enhance overall well-being.

Herbal Support for Reproductive Health: For men interested in optimizing reproductive health and fertility, herbal remedies can offer support for sperm quality and motility. Herbs such as maca root, tribulus terrestris, and fenugreek have been traditionally used to support male reproductive function, increase sperm count and motility, and improve overall fertility. Consuming herbal supplements or teas containing these herbs can help enhance reproductive health and optimize fertility.

Conclusion: In this chapter, we have explored a variety of herbal remedies and practices for supporting men's health and vitality. By incorporating herbs that address specific concerns such as prostate health, hormonal balance, erectile function, stress management, and reproductive health into your daily routine, you can promote men's health naturally. Experiment with different herbs and formulations to find what works best for you, and prioritize self-care as an essential component of your holistic wellness journey as a man. With the gentle support of herbal medicine, you can navigate the unique challenges and transitions of masculinity with vitality and resilience.

Chapter 15: Herbal Remedies for Children's Health

In this chapter, we explore the gentle and effective use of herbal remedies to support children's health and well-being. Children's bodies are still developing, and they may be more sensitive to conventional medications, making herbal medicine a valuable option for addressing common childhood ailments and promoting overall wellness. Let's delve into a variety of herbs and practices aimed at supporting children's health:

Understanding Children's Health: Children's health encompasses a wide range of physical, emotional, and developmental concerns, influenced by factors such as genetics, environment, and lifestyle. From minor illnesses such as colds and digestive issues to more serious conditions like allergies and behavioral challenges, children's health needs vary at different stages of development. Understanding the unique needs of children's health is essential for providing effective and nurturing care.

Gentle Herbs for Common Childhood Ailments: Herbal remedies offer gentle and natural solutions for addressing common childhood ailments such as coughs, colds, fevers, and digestive issues. Herbs such as chamomile, elderberry, and lemon balm have soothing and immune-boosting properties that can help alleviate symptoms and support the body's natural healing processes. Using herbal teas, syrups, or tinctures made from these herbs can provide relief from discomfort and promote recovery from illness.

Herbal Support for Immune Health: Supporting a child's immune system is essential for preventing illness and promoting overall well-being. Herbs such as echinacea, astragalus, and elderberry have immune-enhancing properties that can help strengthen the body's natural defenses and reduce the risk of infections. Incorporating immune-boosting herbs into a child's diet or supplement regimen can help support immune health and reduce the frequency and severity of illnesses.

Herbal Remedies for Digestive Comfort: Children may experience digestive issues such as constipation, diarrhea, or stomachaches from time to time. Herbal remedies such as ginger, fennel, and peppermint have carminative and digestive properties that can help soothe upset stomachs, alleviate gas and bloating, and promote healthy digestion. Offering herbal teas or gentle herbal remedies to children can help ease digestive discomfort and support gastrointestinal health.

Herbal Remedies for Skin Irritations: Children's sensitive skin may be prone to irritations such as rashes, insect bites, or minor cuts and scrapes. Herbal remedies such as calendula, plantain, and lavender have soothing and healing properties that can help relieve itching, reduce inflammation, and promote skin repair. Using herbal salves, creams, or infused oils containing these herbs can provide gentle and effective relief for children's skin irritations.

Safety Considerations and Dosage Guidelines: When using herbal remedies for children, it's essential to prioritize safety and follow appropriate dosage guidelines. Start with low doses and observe for any adverse reactions or allergies. Consult with a qualified herbalist or healthcare provider for personalized recommendations and guidance, especially for infants, young children, or those with underlying health conditions. Use caution when administering herbs to children, and always choose high-quality, organic herbs from reputable sources.

Conclusion: In this chapter, we have explored the gentle and effective use of herbal remedies to support children's health and well-being. By incorporating gentle herbs for common childhood ailments, immune support, digestive comfort, and skin irritations into a child's wellness routine, parents can provide natural and nurturing care for their children. Prioritize safety, follow appropriate dosage guidelines, and consult with healthcare professionals when necessary to ensure the optimal use of herbal remedies for children's health. With the gentle support of herbal medicine, children can thrive and flourish, enjoying optimal health and vitality.

Conclusion:

In this book, we've embarked on a journey through the vast and fascinating world of herbal medicine, exploring the myriad ways in which plants can support health, healing, and well-being. From ancient traditions to modern science, herbal remedies offer gentle and effective solutions for addressing a wide range of health concerns and promoting holistic wellness.

Throughout the chapters, we've delved into the specific applications of herbal medicine for various aspects of health, including:

- **Physical Wellness:** Herbal remedies can support the body's natural healing processes, alleviate symptoms of common ailments, and promote overall physical well-being. Whether it's relieving pain, boosting immunity, or supporting organ function, herbs offer versatile and natural solutions for maintaining health and vitality.

- **Emotional and Mental Health:** Herbs have profound effects on the mind and emotions, offering support for stress management, mood enhancement, and emotional balance. From calming nervine herbs to mood-enhancing botanicals, herbal medicine can help soothe the soul and cultivate inner peace and resilience.

- **Reproductive and Sexual Health:** Herbs play a crucial role in supporting reproductive health and enhancing sexual vitality. Whether it's promoting fertility, balancing hormones, or supporting erectile function, herbal remedies offer gentle and natural solutions for optimizing reproductive and sexual well-being.

- **Children's Health:** Herbal medicine provides gentle and effective support for children's health, addressing common childhood ailments, boosting immune function, and promoting overall well-being. With the right herbs and dosage guidelines, parents can provide natural and nurturing care for their children's health and vitality.

As we conclude our exploration of herbal medicine, it's essential to recognize that while herbs offer valuable therapeutic benefits, they are just one aspect of a holistic approach to health and wellness. Incorporating herbs into a balanced lifestyle that includes healthy nutrition, regular exercise, adequate rest, and stress management is key to achieving optimal well-being.

Furthermore, it's crucial to approach herbal medicine with respect, knowledge, and caution. While herbs are generally safe when used appropriately, it's essential to understand their properties, potential interactions, and contraindications. Consulting with qualified herbalists or healthcare professionals can provide personalized guidance and ensure the safe and effective use of herbal remedies.

Ultimately, herbal medicine offers a profound connection to nature's healing wisdom, empowering individuals to take an active role in their health and well-being. By harnessing the power of plants and incorporating herbal remedies into our lives, we can cultivate vitality, resilience, and harmony with the natural world.

May this book serve as a guide and inspiration on your journey to vibrant health and wellness through the gentle and transformative power of herbal medicine.

Made in United States
Troutdale, OR
05/19/2024

19985517R00066